Table of Contents

Understanding and Overcoming Existential Anxiety: A Therapeutic Approach

1. Introduction to Existential Anxiety

1.1. Definition and Characteristics

1.2. Common Causes

2. Theoretical Frameworks in Understanding Existential Anxiety

2.1. Existentialism

2.2. Terror Management Theory

Existential Anxiety: Symptoms, Treatment, and More

1. Introduction to Existential Anxiety

Existential anxiety can be an unconscious and underlying fear of not having a clear life purpose, but still, as it resides within the unconscious, its exact nature and influence can be difficult to study, diagnose, and heal. Symptoms of existential anxiety include feeling unsatisfied with one's life, isolating oneself, not finding pleasure in things anymore, and waking up at night feeling fear and an impending sense of doom that you can't quite shake. While we live and move on, treating these symptoms is essential in order to help the patient gain back the driver's seat of their life in the long run. Social media, cultural expectations regarding one's personal and documented goals in life, and many other influencers can drive someone within a state of existential depression. In the realm of disapproved environments, some may see a professional. Our approach tries to help deal with the root cause of the disorder and disallows it from manifesting in various physical and mentally disapproved states, in order to comply with these necessities as best as possible.

In this essay, we are going to be studying existential anxiety. We aim to look at the symptoms of existential anxiety, its causes and influencing factors, the cultural background and the healthy nature of this form of anxiety, the impact existential anxiety might have on various populations, and the different ways in which it can be treated. Although he writes using a highly personal lexicon, some of the aspects of our essay are influenced by the psychology of Swiss psychiatrist Carl Gustav Jung (1875–1961), from a synopsis given by a psychological resource called "VeryWellMind". Some of the advice given is attributed to Carl Jung, while the explanations and the general theory had been offered by the same article.

2. Understanding Existential Anxiety

The roots of existential anxiety are multifactorial. Heredity plays a part, as do the specific conditioning experiences that impacted a person from their earliest days. These kinds of experiences make up the content of terror for any given individual. Another factor contributing to existential anxiety is the recognition that no knowledge is ever complete or absolutely certain, and so all knowledge (including scientific knowledge) is necessarily in part a leap of faith. Thus, all "knowledge" is partially belief, and belief is only the logical content of a passionate commitment to a "truth" that will always involve some degree of self-deception. Sudden awareness of the role of faith in knowledge is terrifying for many people because it threatens to undermine all notions of truth and meaning. Failure to hold this connection away is likely to cause a person to slip into an abyss of doubt.

"Existential anxiety" refers to a persistent dread regarding death, freedom, isolation, and a meaningless existence. While this dread is most intense in times of crisis, it is always present in the form of a background dread or fear. Existential anxiety is not a symptom of more superficial personal or cultural malaise, nor is it a direct result of personal problems. Instead, existential anxiety has deep roots that stem from the human condition itself. Existentialists believe that, to varying degrees, everyone has this dread, though most people spend much of their lives distracting themselves from it or denying it. This position is grounded in empirical studies showing that commitment and love-life issues are intertwined and that the way in which people experience anxiety is tied to their core values and sense of purpose. Two people could experience the same trauma, for example, and only one might develop an anxiety disorder, depending on their underlying assumptions about life and meaning.

2.1. Definition and Concept

Throughout time, many people have turned to religion for comfort. It provides specific answers to life's big questions and a promise of immortality and eternal meaning and purpose. For many people, the thought of there not being a bigger plan or a bigger system can be unsettling. We're born, we die, and that's it. The thought of going in that direction can fuel existential anxiety in a big way. Furthermore, it's often accompanied by a belief in the randomness and capriciousness of the universe. Some existentialists believe that everything happens by chance. This may not always be about spirituality, though. For some, existential anxiety may arise from an overwhelming feeling of failure to create a life worth living and disappointments about one's purpose or destiny not panning out.

Existential anxiety is a form of anxiety that is based on concerns about big, sometimes profound, philosophical or spiritual issues. It can be one of the most difficult forms of anxiety for individuals to work through because of the very nature of existential and life-and-death type questioning that is at the root of it. Existentialism as a philosophical paradigm is based on an offshoot of atheism and, to some extent, nihilism. It places an emphasis on free will and the ability of the individual to create his or her own sense of meaning in life, apart from outside religious, social, or moral prescriptions. In general, it promotes the idea that there is no inherent meaning in life, that life itself is absurd, and that meaning and purpose must be self-created.

Existential Anxiety: What is it?

2.2. Causes and Triggers

With that said, many other potential causes and triggers have been linked to the development of existential anxiety. A few, in particular, include feelings of isolation, loneliness, and a fear of being alone, a general lack of identity or personality, and an inability to find oneself – at least in some capacity – and a general uncertainty or fear about the future or what lies beyond the grave. These things are common in people who experience an existential crisis and share all the same feelings of fear and despair as the crisis itself can muster. A feeling of having wasted one's life and its inherent opportunities is also often cited as a potential cause for existential anxiety, be it due to loss or feelings of guilt and regret. Tragedy and trauma are other common events in one's life that are directly linked to existential crises, though they haven't been associated as much as other potential triggers when it comes to anxiety disorders.

While having an existential crisis can bring existential anxiety, they're not one and the same: experiencing an existential crisis doesn't guarantee that one will develop anxiety disorder, and having a diagnosed existential anxiety disorder does not inherently mean you are in an existential crisis. Nevertheless, existential crises often contribute to anxiety and are a common trigger for anxiety disorders of all kinds. This stands to reason since such crises can bring about extreme stress, fear, depression, and all of the other emotions that can gradually develop into an anxiety disorder over time. We know that existential anxiety can develop as a result of this particular event because of its association with the development of generalized anxiety disorders and similar conditions.

3. Symptoms of Existential Anxiety

Emotional Signs: The former tends to reveal existential anxiety symptoms in a more straightforward manner. Many individuals, either because of their own existential reflection or because that of another, will confront the malaise and depression of reality. When contemplating our own insignificance in a world replete with cosmic horror, the absurd repetition of existence reveals that an individual can never truly move past the suffering. These truths can make life lamentable, to the point where enjoyment feels somewhat sweeter, yet no less amusing, than pain. It is from these ideas that existential angst begins showing itself, but somehow still manages to twist itself back into a feeling entirely different to the one expected.

Certain species of birds seem to have an awareness of their own mortality. They show characteristics associated with human emotions like grief when a fellow bird dies. What these birds go through and how they go through it is something that could be deemed paralyzing and oversensitive. The fact that reminders of death can hasten this feeling serves as a hollow swipe against the perception that sensitivity with regards to a particular subject is a rather praiseworthy and useful trait. Such sensitivities lead an individual to experience the symptoms of existential anxiety, which are associated with the many symptoms of clinical anxiety yet are nonetheless related. One can divide the symptoms of existential anxiety into emotional and physical signs.

3.1. Physical Symptoms

Our bodies often respond to anxiety and fear with the fight or flight response. With existential anxiety, there's no immediate threat you can flee from or diffuse with physical action. So, the adrenaline created by being in a constant state of fear may produce feelings of restlessness, impotent anger, or a sense of powerlessness. Existential anxiety and the resulting physical symptoms can end up feeding off each other. It becomes a vicious cycle, with your mind and body reinforcing one another's symptoms. This pattern is hard to break. Cognitive-behavioural therapy (CBT) has shown promise in helping the body recognise and combat anxiety before the symptoms become overwhelming.

Existential anxiety can cause both emotional and physical symptoms. Physical symptoms may include fatigue, nausea, shortness of breath, dizziness or lightheadedness, vertigo, rapid heart rate, chest pain, sweating, gastrointestinal distress, tremors, muscle tension or spasms, headache or migraine, insomnia or sleeping too much, chronic pain, and chronic illness. If you're experiencing any of these symptoms, it's important to see a healthcare provider to rule out the presence of any medical conditions.

Existential anxiety affects individuals emotionally and physically. It can cause an intense dread that you're wasting your life. This existential anxiety may spur you to make changes or it might keep you feeling stuck and helpless. Everyone experiences this anxiety differently. If existential anxiety is interfering with your life, it makes sense to seek help.

3.2. Emotional Symptoms

For where is the external cause of the angst, when there is no longer any object at which to direct one's hitherto trained fears and desires? Where is the shaking surface for frail emotion, when it is the very ground of one's existence that is shifting away beneath one's feet? When the fear of a specific event has passed into the fear of the event itself, how is one to proceed? In a very real sense, it is the specifically euphoric and emotionally intense aspect of anxiety over and above softer moods such as worry that defines the existential aspect of one's dread and despair.

A vital clue to the understanding of the root of existential anxiety is present in a key symptom of the condition. While it is true that the individual becomes intimidated, disoriented, and apprehensive of their nature and their future, they are equally overwhelmed by a feeling of meaninglessness and despair. It is the latter symptom, the intrinsic feelings of angst, hopelessness, and dread that is most troubling in the case of existential anxiety.

Existential anxiety, as we have come to understand, involves the fear, disorientation, and disquiet resulting from the confrontation of one's life and one's death. The emotion is indeed a complex blend of psychological unease and philosophical despair.

Overunderstanding the emotions involved in existential anxiety requires a sufficient understanding of what existential anxiety truly is. While we have now discussed both the definition and symptoms of existential anxiety in detail thus far, we haven't inquired into the emotional aspect yet.

4. Impact on Daily Life

Here's a look at how existential anxiety can affect someone's life in various ways. Relationships: Existential anxiety can cause tension in friendships and relationships. When someone's struggling, talking about it with others may not make them feel better. "While discussing existential concerns with supportive individuals can have some benefits, it can also produce negative feelings including fear of judgment and isolation," says Dr. Abdallah. Work: It can be difficult to focus on work-related tasks when feeling consumed by thoughts of meaning and purpose. This sick-of-work feeling can also make someone feel isolated. "In the work environment, people with existential anxiety may feel disconnected with others," adds Dr. Abdallah. Symptoms can be mild to severe, very similar to general anxiety disorder, from mild displaced anxiety and discomfort all the way to severe disruption of daily life and panic attacks. The disorder can be related to anxiety-based issues, such as addiction, depression, or anger.

We all think about existential questions from time to time. It's natural because we're human. But when it starts affecting your quality of life, it becomes a problem. "Existential anxiety can be extremely debilitating," says Dr. Zerkel. "People may have a hard time enjoying life, due to fear of death or fear of lack of purpose and meaning. They may avoid thinking about the questions to avoid anxiety or, conversely, they may be consumed by thoughts about these questions." Existential anxiety can also lead a person to question ways of life that they used to value. Someone who always answered that they were "carefree" and "just went with the flow" may suddenly start getting consumed by questions and fears. "Consciousness of the negative side of life can lead them to question things they used to take for granted," explains Dr. Abdallah.

5. Diagnosis and Assessment

Person-Centered interviewing: This type of assessment uses open-ended prompts for individuals to provide "storytelling" type responses about their background, heritage, goals, values, interests, and activities, among other subjects. This insight can help mental health professionals in the diagnosis of existential anxiety and the development of a broader treatment plan that lines up with an individual's beliefs and values.

Comorbidity: Anxiety, including existential anxiety, often occurs alongside other mental health conditions. A thorough assessment will therefore try to look at comorbidity by evaluating for other anxiety disorders, depression, substance use, and others.

Checklist: Sometimes mental health professionals will use a checklist to gather information about a person's level of distress and symptoms related to anxiety. This symptom checklist may ask someone how often certain feelings occur. Clinicians may also ask someone about factors contributing to the anxiety, including certain stressors, as well as lifestyle and coping strategies.

Making a diagnosis of existential anxiety can be difficult, as existential anxiety is not a formally recognized diagnosis. It is important for individuals struggling with existential anxiety to reach out to qualified mental health professionals for assessment and not attempt to self-diagnose. That said, there are certain assessment approaches that clinicians may use to evaluate the type of anxiety with which someone is struggling, including existential anxiety.

6. Treatment Approaches

2. Medications. Talk therapy isn't the only way to combat symptoms of existential anxiety. Some individuals may also find help through medication. Typically, doctors prescribe anxiolytics, such as selective serotonin reuptake inhibitors (SSRIs), and benzodiazepines (Ativan and Valium). However, these medications target symptoms, not causes. Instead, SSRIs are prescribed for symptoms of generalized anxiety disorder (GAD), but exposure therapy and/or CBT is considered the best treatment. If needed, your doctor is the best source for recommendations and prescriptions for anxiety-related medications. However, the ultimate goal is to treat the root cause. An expert in existentialism has a greater depth in providing effective psychotherapy. Furthermore, doctors can suggest GAD medications like anxiolytics or antidepressants for people with serious symptoms. However, they often work best in conjunction with a variety of therapies, not just by themselves.

1. Therapy and counseling. Cognitive-behavioral therapy (CBT), as well as emotion-focused therapy and existential analysis, are common treatments for people coping with existential anxiety. Although not as widely used as CBT, mindfulness-based therapies may have a role in increasing a person's sense of awareness. Exploring any past traumas through therapy can also provide useful information about your current thought patterns. Evidence also exists that meeting with a priest, rabbi, imam, or another religious leader can help.

Your ability to overcome existential anxiety may depend, in part, on its severity and how it's impacting your life. Several treatment approaches may be used to help alleviate symptoms associated with existential anxiety. These include:

6.1. Therapy and Counseling

The primary method for dealing with existential anxiety is existential therapy. Existential therapy is a philosophical approach that recognizes the actuality of human consciousness and their existence so highly that it is used for therapeutic purposes. In addition to this, while the feeling of anxiety itself is what a therapist is called in to assist with, most people do not primarily go to therapy with the goal of treating existential anxiety. More often than not, individuals go to therapy with an initial problem of anxiety that they believe the existential anxiety is a side effect of. In this case, therapy would be used to address the current, most pressing issue and changes the person has made in their life since then. This change is specifically what some therapists who can take a public health approach to counseling and utilize weekly groups to help teach others how to identify and address negative emotional impacts may also further reduce the prevalence of existential anxiety itself, as well as symptoms like it, on a community level.

The experience of existential anxiety alone can be enough to set off a seemingly endless set of additional symptoms and side effects. One particularly effective way to handle an existential crisis is through the support of a mental health professional. A therapist can help provide the necessary coping skills, strategies, and processing to help you address your deepest fears and unknowns.

6.2. Medication

Pharmacotherapy: Antidepressants (e.g., Selective serotonin reuptake inhibitors: fluoxetine, sertraline, paroxetine, citalopram, escitalopram). The serotonin and norepinephrine reuptake inhibitor venlafaxine is an effective treatment that may be used for existential anxiety, as well as depression and anxiety as co-occurring presentations. Antidepressants may assist individuals to develop increased tolerance of existential anxiety, which at times may aid an increase in coping mechanism skills developed, improved coping, and reduced resistance to negative emotions. Improvement is noted in sleep, mood, and ability to cope with the anxiety or distress. Some reports from the practice and case reports note a reduced intensity of existential-related anxiety and depression following prescription, but the existing studies typically have used only measures of general anxiety or anxiety symptoms with an anxious presentation. Thus, it is difficult to be confident about the overall treatment approach. Antidepressants are mainly prescribed alongside therapy to increase the speed and effectiveness of the individual's response, especially when a short course of medication is proposed.

Medication Table: Medications used in the treatment of existential anxiety Medication class Specific medication Which presentations appear to worsen or improve with this medication Selective serotonin reuptake inhibitors (SSRIs) Fluoxetine, sertraline, paroxetine, citalopram, escitalopram TBD Serotonin and norepinephrine reuptake inhibitors (SNRIs) Venlafaxine TBD Tricyclic antidepressants St. John's Wort TBD Second generation antipsychotics Quetiapine, olanzapine, risperidone, clozapine TBD Other (e.g., mood stabilizers, anti-anxiety, or 'hypnotic' medications) Mirtazapine TBD

Treatment & Management

7. Self-Help Strategies

7. Reflection and inquiry: Liverpool-based psychotherapist Ferimer states that as a way of exploring their existential anxieties, people should allow themselves to sit in contemplation and embrace genuine curiosity. By inquiring openly, they can make new meanings and interpretations. At the same time, inquiring into why they start to feel anxious can be useful for those who are experiencing negative thoughts around the future and what it might hold for them. This will help them to understand more about what is contributing to their worries.

6. Journaling: Taking time to journal your thoughts on existential crises or even spending time journaling in a stream of consciousness writing practice can be therapeutic and help you to feel your experience more deeply.

5. Values, purpose, and self-care: Take the time to contemplate your unique values and purpose in life. Create routines that revolve around taking care of yourself to rebalance your life and get re-grounded.

4. Mindfulness and meditation: Better understand your emotions with meditation. Use Schwalbe's meditation technique, which helps to focus on the answers to some essential questions: Who am I? Where am I going? Who do I want to be while I'm in the outer world?

3. Practicing bravery: Allow yourself to confront your fears and overcome your dislike, fear, or limited knowledge of

things that create anxiety and doubt in your life. This can increase your self-confidence. You can also use CBT approaches such as gradual exposure to do so.

2. Coping and courage: Engage with friends, family members, or colleagues to practice courage and seek meaning. Share your feelings about your doubts and worries to help you cope with anxiety.

1. Mindfulness: Practice mindfulness to focus on the present moment and reduce worry. You might include breathing exercises or body scans to release physical tension and help you relax.

7.1. Mindfulness and Meditation Techniques

According to research, transpersonal psychology suggests that mindfulness and meditation practices are effective for facilitating development, adding well-being, and reducing stress waves. "Scientifically validated, mindfulness-based stress reduction (MBSR) programs offer an integrated learning experience, consisting of take-home technique recordings, classes focused on physical movement, frequent meditation breaks, teacher-led discussion, and assigned homework sessions," according to the UMass Medical School Center for Mindfulness. Some of these courses include hatha or vinyasa yoga, walking meditation, and body scan. Mindfulness or vipassana insight meditation is also practiced during the courses. As part of the CAMS process, many therapists and clients incorporate a mindfulness meditation practice, with an emphasis on breath awareness. More sophisticated meditations, such as Loving Kindness (Metta-Bhavana), Tonglen, Mindful Eating, and Mani, are often part of Tibetan, Zen, or mindfulness practices. Dr. Paul Gilbert suggests engaging in Loving Kindness meditations that focus on empathy for others' suffering and self-care practices.

Immersing oneself in mindfulness meditation can be beneficial, as it can help a person develop new ways of coping with psychological discomfort. Eckhart Tolle maintains that "mindfulness represents more than just a specific meditation technique; it also represents a combination of concentration and meditation. Block out the world and love instead." It also brings an individual to a sensory, present awareness, ideally free from preconceived thoughts and fears. For those who open themselves to the experience, body awareness recorded by the nervous system and emotional release are part of the adventure. Here are some simple ways to incorporate a mindfulness/meditation practice into one's life, according to the work of Dr. Aaron Beck. It is possible to meditate while remaining true to everyday life.

7.2. Journaling and Reflection

When have you felt this way in the past? (the recent past or even in your childhood) Did any specific event(s) come before those feelings? Is there any chance those events or similar experiences occur again? How can you plan ahead to address those emotions? There is validation in seeing the progression from "oh, that's what I'm feeling" to "tell me about it", as reflected in your journal entries. Could journaling be a coping mechanism for the feelings brought up through introspection? If your anxiety (or any mental health) begins to feel unmanageable and makes daily living difficult/unsafe, consider reaching out for help.

Remember to ask yourself why and keep your entries organized with headers or bullet points. Reflection often works in tandem with journaling. A theme in therapy is the power of introspection (or self-reflection). A moment of self-awareness might come with unpleasant emotions, but over time being open to what you learn will allow you to understand yourself more deeply and manage how you feel. It can also help prevent emotional outbursts, though compartmentalization is not a goal. Instead, by expressing your feelings, you can make it easier to head them off at the pass before they explode or result in a different physical, emotional, or mental health "side effect".

Journaling may seem like a small undertaking, but it can have powerful effects on mental health and well-being and might even reduce symptoms of mild to moderate anxiety. Writing is more than a form of self-expression; it can be a real-life, doctor-recommended anxiety treatment. Journaling about your thoughts and emotions can help to identify patterns and discover the root causes of your emotional anguish; keep those running through your head from feeling so encompassing and monumental.

8. Coping with Existential Anxiety in Relationships

It is possible for someone with existential anxiety to be going through a relationship filled with anxiety and thus unhealthy for the couple in how they experience the fears, thoughts, and anxieties. They often fear being perceived as clingy and avoid discussing their existential anxiety with their partner or therapists because of the anxiety of being left by those who have actually decided to be in their lives and accept them for who they are. Nonetheless, by addressing existential anxiety, one can cope better and may find that their relationship improves. The following are some of these coping strategies. Dealing with experiencing existential anxiety may be done alone or with the help of a therapist who is beyond willing to help. The counseling that sooner a person goes to counseling, the more likely they are to regain trust, talk, and communicate in their relationship. This, in turn, allows the partner to help the individual suffering from existential anxiety.

Coping Mechanisms

Dealing with existential anxiety can cause a person's perception to change in such a way that they see the larger problems in life and how they relate to themselves on a personal level. This often forces a turning point in relationships as many people do not understand the complications of living with existential anxiety. They include how life is meaningless, how they are choosing to live, etc. All of these factors shape a general existence and "being in the world". So, how should we cope with existential anxiety in relationships?

9. Existential Anxiety in Different Age Groups

Anxiety at all ages can manifest through physical symptoms. In children, this often appears as acting "new" or younger than their actual age, bedwetting, and becoming clingy. They also can experience existential depression. Teens struggle more with the purpose of life or what gives life meaning. That can manifest as intense feelings of not wanting to be here or questioning if life is worth continuing. Teens can be more consumed with the thwarting of potential, such as failing at something that means a lot to them. In early adulthood, individuals focus more on situational driven anxiety such as college, finding a job, making friends, settling down and finding a partner. When existential anxiety is present, many fear missing opportunities and leading a meaningless existence. They often are competing with others and worry about being left behind. As adults age, existential anxiety in the form of terror of death and dying increases for many as their health declines. Younger adults often worry about their existential suffering and talk about how they don't want to be a burden on their families. Adults worry about how this will impact their own and their families' quality of life. For older adults, death and dying are a part of the natural life-cycle. The focus shifts to legacy, how will I be remembered by my family and in my communities? In the first half of life, people are busy mostly with values related to performance and striving toward accomplishments. In later life, it is more about intrinsic values, such as love, friendship, generosity, and how can I help others since older adults have likely had meaningful work experiences and have made their contributions to society.

Existential anxiety is a common human experience that can affect people of all ages. As each age group progresses through the developmental stage, the anxieties may manifest differently. This article will provide an overview of the existential anxiety experienced and how it presents in children, adolescents, adults, and older adults.

9.1. Children and Adolescents

In evaluative terms, such models suggest to parents and professionals that the correct way to deal with a child making such statements is not to reinforce them through over-reaction and unnecessary medical intervention, but, conversely, not to dismiss or deride them either; rather, professionals and parents should remain reassuring but open and non-adversarial in their responses. Regardless of the category of death anxiety presented during illness, temporary visits to the existential limit may still occur. In these situations, the reality of life-threatening illness impinges upon patients who are mentally prepared to explore the existential pole of existence. For some patients experiencing deep existential anxiety, this is the first time that they have been confronted by any psychosocial or psychological consideration. In effect, in the NHS, the questions were post-facto and unintentional.

As mentioned before, the phenomenological perspective emphasizes the ongoing need for continued self-constitution in confrontation with issues not yet fully built into the ego. This is related to different anxiety dynamics at different developmental stages. Regarding children and adolescents, they have awareness of the vulnerability and danger inherent in being new to the world and needing protection. They understand that they are functioning within a universe over which they have little control and are most often necessary to arrive at an initial understanding of the prevalence and spontaneous appearance of the early "founderal" variety. It is very often the context of life-changing events such as the death of a grandparent, the birth of a new sibling, or starting school that precipitate such founderal experiences in childhood, just as the birth of a first child or the prospect of becoming a parent may do so in adulthood. In children, there have been further suggestions that a founderal variety of death anxiety may, however, show greater cognitive maturity and referentiality.

9.2. Adults and Older Adults

Patients continue to experience existential anxiety and fear of death, concerns about the immediate future, and the threat of the uncontrolled in the late phase of treatment for cancer. Individuals with neurodegenerative conditions such as idiopathic Parkinson's disease report existential anxiety linked to their somatic symptoms and medications. Of patients with Huntington's disease, 59% state that awareness of the diagnosis results in symptoms of enormous existential anxiety. First-time nursing home residents are confronted with a level of freedom of choice regarding food, religion, schedule, and activities, which can lead to high existential anxiety. Eighty-two percent of older adults report that existential anxiety related to concerns about communicating preferences for need-to-know ethics. People with Alzheimer's disease report loss of control of many functions, such as driving the car and decision-making, to be situations mainly associated with anxiety. Residents in nursing homes report extreme existential anxiety in cases of financial uncertainty and the inability to prepare for old age, containing thoughts of a great loss of self-determination and a lifelong apprehension of old age handled through complete denial of the circumstances.

Older Adults

Existential anxiety has been considered a universal experience to a greater extent than other emotions. Older adults see existential anxiety as an emotional part of the aging process, while adults perceive it as the outcome of certain events or living conditions. Existential anxiety associated with older adults is recognized as conscious or repressed, inhibitive or constructive, and linked with coherence or attitude in environmental adaptation.

Adulthood

10. Existential Anxiety and Mental Health Disorders

Comorbidities are complex and unique to each person. Some people may experience mild existential anxiety off and on, whereas others may have more severe, chronic anxiety. Therapy and sometimes medication, such as antidepressants or anti-anxiety medication, are common ways to combat these issues. Cheaning says "evidence-based therapies used to treat a variety of mental health disorders, such as cognitive behavioral therapy (CBT), have also been shown to help alleviate the symptoms of existential anxiety. Existential anxiety exists on a spectrum that is linked with numerous other mental health disorders." Much of the time, she adds, people may find that their existential anxiety starts to fade as their mental health improves.

At times, existential anxiety can be severe enough to affect daily life. Whether you already have a mental illness or are living with existential anxiety alone, it's important to seek support from a mental health professional. When a person is dealing with a mental health disorder - like anxiety or depression - existential anxiety can also be present. Existential anxiety can heighten the symptoms of other mental health issues. For example, a person living with general anxiety may find that worries about the future trigger an existential tailspin. Mental health disorders and existential anxiety can impact each other. People who have lived through trauma or are dealing with a chronic illness may naturally struggle with questions like "why me?"

11. Existential Anxiety in the Workplace

Employers have an obligation to reduce harm or suffering of apprentices where reasonably possible. Employers must be prepared to assist employees to identify and address feelings of work-related existential anxiety. Sensitive ethical responsibility and professionalism demand that managers make special effort to discern expressions of existential anxiety that might lie hidden behind traditional symptoms of stress. Workplace safety legislation in several jurisdictions now sets out that organizational interventions may be required in some cases to prevent or manage work-related stress. In workplaces where adhering to daily routines and procedures with little variation is a hallmark, or for those with little access to the natural world, the link between a lack of control over major life concerns and depression, despair, or unease may not be difficult to see. Identifying those aspects of working life that increase a sense of unease and despair, and removing or mitigating them may be one practical step towards having a life that is meaningful.

The experience of existential anxiety often spills over into—or is reinforced by—an individual's workplace. As we explored earlier, workplace norms often demand people hide signs of existential anxiety. In many industries, rather than an admittance of difficulty or suffering, the appearance of calm and control are expected. Moreover, many people fear that discussing meaning at work is unprofessional or that others will assume they operate below desirable efficiency benchmarks. Despite the potential for existential anxiety to compromise attention span, judgment, and confidence, many employers expect workers to keep their attention in the present moment, make the best possible decisions, and be a team player, come what may. It would be presumptuous to presume an individual's deep feelings and requiring them to remain hidden could be in accordance with sound ethical principles.

12. Existential Anxiety and Spirituality

Existential anxiety is the anxiety that derives from the tension emanating from existential concerns. This anxiety is to be distinguished from mere natural anxiety, for instance the kind of teenage angst that comes from hormone surges. Existential anxiety is a kind of result of laying back and examining one's life, in which one can come to realize that people dedicate their lives to often illusory states, there is no intrinsic purpose injectable into life, and in the grand scheme of the cosmos lives of earth-dwellers are of no cosmic importance. It is reported that people, especially as they approach death, realize these facts, resulting in an often gut-wrenching anxiety. Existential anxiety also appears in some forms of psychotherapy, as a result of people's resistance to open up and speak to their therapists. Identified in all these descriptions is a deep, antsy fear of the unknown: of death, of what lies beyond one's illusions, or how oneself will be at the end of the day true.

Christian S. Chan, a Buddhist, offers a detailed Buddhist account of existential anxiety. This leads into an exploration of the relationship between existential anxiety and spirituality. According to the overview provided here, some utilize their spirituality to cope with their existential anxiety. Others, however, are so anxious and petrified that their spirituality is inhibited. This section is relevant for understanding not only the spiritual dimensions of coping with existential anxiety, but the link between spirituality and psychological well-being. It is also significant in addressing the suspicious response to Coulehan's idea that meditation can help doctors cope with existential anxiety.

13. Research and Studies on Existential Anxiety

Perhaps unlike most other disorders in the DSM-5, very little information exists on existential anxiety. Fillippetti et al. have proposed an interesting distinction between the two ideas of "existential anxiety" and "anxiety tied to mortality." For a more general or existential discussion, this scenario is the instructor's desired make-believe, and the term "existential anxiety" is the most accurate identifier for that idea. Fortunately, a smattering of Massachusetts-based community programs has been studied to some degree. One such program is Satsang Saurabh, a free mental health community program reportedly created "in response to existential distress related to the global pandemic." Facilitated in Hindi via Zoom, the program was started by three first-generation Indian immigrants who are—also—healers in "task-oriented professions of engineering, technology, and science.

A categorically systematic laundry list lays mostly dormant, although an existential anxiety scale of some sort may exist. Scattered studies on the topic focus on (1) how existential anxiety relates to other constructs and (2) therapy or community programs that may help to mitigate existential anxiety. Assuming such a list is developed, the first goal ought to be identifying the enfants terribles among the items to ensure that the list is avoiding circular arguments about the essence of existential anxiety. For that purpose, refer to Yalom, if not here, then at least in the work itself. Additional reading assignments are best conveyed at the introductory discussion.

14. Future Directions in Existential Anxiety Research

15. Conclusion and Key Takeaways

Diagnosed in its broadest sense, existential anxiety is the anxiety of our response to life and reveals our subjective association with the worlds and spaces we traverse. This anxiety reflects a profound type of suffering of our surroundings and ourselves, as well as the loss of care and solicitude that logos have for us in our world. As a degree of freedom over and above mere biophysical subsistence, existential anxiety should be an object of ethical and pathological concern for healthcare professionals who engage with patients within an acute care psychiatric setting. It is clear that the world is both indifferent and available for the existential and anxiety disordered individuals, that death is the primary concern, and the subject is a perspective being limited by its transcendence within its world. While we are excessively open to the world and others, we can only present this world dressed in our being and the terminally ill are denied this possibility. The individual's priority of death, anxiety, and care allow themselves to be interpreted by considering the relevant form of being-il in question.

In this essay, I have examined the concept of existential anxiety and aimed to outline its features, root causes, and scope. The essay has been divided into three main components, bridging three distinct sections. The first section sought to carve out a working definition of existential anxiety, unearthing the two-component framework through which it becomes intelligible. It was illuminated that existential anxiety is, at its core, a distress of our subjective association with our surroundings, while diagnosing existential anxiety as a suffering of the totality of existence. Section two discussed the root causes of existential anxiety: knowing of our death, freedom, and loss of meaning in life. It was uncovered that this anxiety is normally painful but is a meaningful and healthy component of being human. Finally, section three sought to illustrate a few of the myriad concrete manifestations of existential anxiety and interrogated its phenomenological scope, concluding that existential anxiety is universal while the particular shape it takes can be individualized.

Understanding and Overcoming Existential Anxiety: A Therapeutic Approach

1. Introduction to Existential Anxiety

Finally, in keeping with the existential philosophical tradition, a movement that had passionately warned us about the potential psychic injury our psychology can do to our being on this planet behind the veil and experience of deathness, an indifferent universe, they called forth in "Being and Nothingness" the aching vertigo of emptiness and meaninglessness, of anxiety in the face of nihility, ennui as they attributed to the young man with the inkpot. It can be a lonely and deadening condition when one lives among people who do not really share the meaning and passion of your desire.

Our early work suggests that existential anxiety isn't a monolithic entity but is characterizable as a frustration that we cannot realize the being that we have set our hopes on and, in our hopes, to become and experience with it requited love. There are four main ingredients of this recipe for existential anxiety: 1) Longing and Deficiency; 2) A lack of confidence in ourselves and our ability to create our existence; 3) A quest for meaning, a purpose of existence. These, our first tentative psychological descriptions of the four main components of existential anxiety, focus around four interconnected, common yet negative aspects, firstly that of the Freudian unconscious, the realm out of which desire flows, secondly that of power, the lack of which generates lack of confidence in self and others, thirdly that of meaning and purpose, about the desire to see that we have made a difference, that life is worth living and that the purpose was worth the suffering.

Existential anxiety is fearfulness par excellence since it doesn't have a concrete object but is rather directed at nonexistence - a state which cannot be conceptualized. In contrast to the neurotic, who fears only certain dangers, the fearful person is afraid of everything, and hence also of nothing, since the most fearful thing of all is the absence of fear - in this case, so-called existential angst, an empty, cloudy feeling, which is monotonous and oppressive: the feeling of the meaninglessness of life, of the terror of existence. It is the feeling that we have nothing in life to hope for and are groundlessly hopeful.

One of the most intriguing problems in the philosophy of psychiatry is how to understand and deal with existential psychopathology, such as existential anxiety and angst. Typically, existential anxiety is thought to be a general term that denotes the encompassing anxious mood - a mood that entirely determines our attitude to what it is to exist. More specifically, it names the fear of nonexistence, which is based on the feeling that our existence is threatened or can, does, or will come to nothing.

1.1. Definition and Characteristics

Existential anxiety is a unique type of anxiety, one that perhaps stems from a different nature than the rest. While all forms of anxiety are only tentatively rooted in reality, to an extent, existential anxiety is, in some sense or another, deeply ingrained. Intrinsically tied to the essence of man, existential anxiety contains several components. First, there is a futility and dreadfulness to discovering that the cultural values swallow us whole. Because culture is a type of anodyne against the irrational terror of life, to realize that these trappings hold no power in and of themselves to save us neutralizes the value of the culture, theories, and individual lifestyles in a Nietzschean sense. In this weighting and measuring of all existence, we also realize that our human sentiments and connubiality do not reduce this grand cruelty one bit. The finding that our medications do not work causes immense anxiety, particularly in modern times. It destroys the relative sense of comfort that we derive from living our lives running on faith and trust, permitting us to ignore the sheer senselessness of our pursuits—the essential worth that is never attainable—and instead, to defend ourselves against the world by living in such a way that we live forever.

The experience of humanity is one that brings with it ineluctable questions of meaning and value. Confronted with the reality of our own uncertain futures, most of us experience particularly stressful periods that prompt us to seek meaning, authenticity, and a truth that is truly our own. Existential anxiety, also referred to as existential dread, can be described as a presence of dread imbued with psychological distress as we face the bare bones of the human condition, particularly the realization that life is a long death march with no end but to cease existence, not to mention that one day, the vast majority of us will be forgotten altogether. This is one facet of the existential dilemma, which is a unique sort of suffering that results from the sudden and overwhelming confrontation with an existential reality that transcends human emotion and capacity to reconcile.

1.2. Common Causes

Isolation can take the form of subjective loneliness and has been well-discussed by Kierkegaard, Tillich, May, Yalom, and others as being the most profound form of isolation to the individual. It can also be the result of a specific disruption in the degree to which we are related to the Other. Similarly, in both cases economic relatedness, compromises to our personhood can take the form of role conflicts or major life transitions that may induce an identity crisis. Executives who are reengineering corporations, force downsizing, and collapsing functions also demonstrate more existential anxiety.

While the nature of existential anxiety is complex and multifaceted, some of the common causes of this form of anxiety or distress include a climate or environment of mortality preoccupation or awareness. The danger of death and unknown that existentialism invites as the realization of our finiteness also applies when our potential is not being realized or we feel existentially isolated. For example, any degree of isolation can also make us more aware of the suffering and potential for loneliness that accompanies layers of relating. This concept has been confirmed from both qualitative interview-level results from researchers like Fontaine and the quantitative MedStat reports weeks before the economic downturn of 2007-2008.

2. Theoretical Frameworks in Understanding Existential Anxiety

Terror management theory (TMT) appears to be a combination of existentialism and cognitive social psychology. It has been conducting numerous experiments in the last two decades on this topic. TMT, developed by three researchers Jeff Greenberg, Tom Pyszcynski, and Sheldon Solomon, has exerted an enormous influence on social psychology. Craig (2008) has said that "The contribution shows that the terror of the meaninglessness of life can have a great impact on human activity, and even serves as the basis for group self-creation and self-management activities leading to the social organization." It is seen that this terror plays an important role in culture, including religion, philosophy, politics, and art. A concrete action plan organized to avoid such anxiety is known as terrorism management theory. According to TMT, the potential for or the incidence of existential anxiety, caused basically by the awareness of the inevitability of human death and of one's vulnerability, has universal and personal dimensions. Also, TMT focuses on attempts at threat mitigation – psychological structures that are activated by stimulus that poses a signal of potential anxiety. It results operationally, TMT researchers recognize that fear of death motivates people to look for ways to gain self-esteem or to seek symbolic immortality. Alternatively, individuals might employ different strategies for reducing mortality concerns.

Theoretical frameworks that help in understanding existential anxiety are existentialism and terror management theory. Existentialism, as a philosophical and psychoanalytic system, believes that existential anxiety is a part and parcel of the existence of an individual. It is the awareness of the absolute aloneness and the absurdity of existence. It is not a result of lack of some biological need or due to some kind of mishap or frustration in life. Whenever one begins to wonder about the meaning and purpose of life and death, he has to face anxiety. Søren Kierkegaard was the first one who used the nationality detailed analysis of anxiety. He gave a detailed account of anxiety's distinctive physical symptoms, such as dizziness and the sense of having a sinking feeling. It signifies a "nothingness of the spirit".

2.1. Existentialism

Central to existentialist philosophy is the idea that, in the absence of absolute meaning, humans must create value in their individual lives. When there is no inherent purpose or meaning to human life, this gives rise to large-scale meaninglessness or absurdity. Another dimension along which existentialism might help us to understand existential anxiety is the concern with authenticity. Reactions to existential threats can reveal aspects of our personalities (e.g., our priorities, what we find threatening) and whether we are acting out of an authentic sense of self or inauthentically. The search for an authentic self is often seen as a key existential task, meaning that difficult questions about human freedom, choice, self-responsibility, and identity are of paramount importance.

Existentialism is a theoretical framework for understanding existential anxiety. Several concepts at the heart of existentialism resonate with the phenomenon of existential anxiety. Many existential thinkers suggest that authentic human existence is fraught with dread or anxiety because of the weight of our freedom. Existentialism holds that individual humans account for their experiences and actions, and it is we who establish what is important in the world. This interconnectedness of freedom, individual responsibility, and identity goes some way to explaining why existential questions and concerns are deeply personal and difficult to discard.

2.2. Terror Management Theory

TMT posits that an awareness of mortality is intrinsic to the human condition. According to the theory, humans' strong drive for self-preservation creates a powerful aversion to death that becomes extremely distressing when confronted with their own mortality. Despite the threat posed by the knowledge of death, however, humans are autonomous beings living in a constantly changing and unpredictable environment. To reduce death anxiety, humans do what they can to manage it. One way that humans manage death anxiety is to be convinced that they are 'important people' who will be positively remembered. Although self-esteem is a crucial part of managing the terror of death, self-esteem can be fragile. If a person invests in achieving and maintaining self-worth via the internalization of symbolically constructed, culturally derived values, then self-threat is likely to naturally occur if the symbols' representations are devalued or rejected.

Ernest Becker (1973) foregrounded the central role that the awareness of the inevitability of mortality has in fueling anxiety, terror, and anger, and proposed it as the common source of almost all human destructiveness. As such, the fear of death has been identified in the existential literature as an important component in existential anxiety, and is explicitly argued to powerfully condition the moment-to-moment anxiety responses of clients in distress elsewhere. Researchers working within 'terror management theory' (TMT) advance this understanding of the role of mortality concerns in fear and anxiety.

3. Effects of Existential Anxiety on Mental Health

Beck, Rush, Shaw, and Emery enumerated a set of cognitive distortions - including catastrophizing, overgeneralization, and personalization - that could cause pain and difficulties. These cognitive distortions can appear with more frequency in anxiety disorders than in depression. Viktor Frankl believed there is a fear of depression that lies behind many lesser fears. Individuals try to run away from death because they are afraid of the pain that may accompany death. This is true of existential anxiety as well. Given such a widespread occurrence, it is not surprising that a host of mental health issues and symptoms can be traced back to existential anxiety. For example, a person might develop an anxiety-related disorder when he/she believes that life must have a purpose, a meaning, and value in order to live it. The mind commands the body to produce that biochemical at once. It gives an immediacy. There is neither time nor need to reflect, to weigh, to appreciate.

Existential anxiety significantly impacts people's personal and professional lives. Self-imposed deadlines and responsibilities levy tremendous pressure on individuals who are already full-to-overflowing with anxiety. There are both intrinsic and extrinsic motivators leading to such pressures. The focus of these pressures is the urgent need to prove to themselves and to others that their existence has a meaning and that it is purposeful. It therefore cheers

us immensely when we are taught the defensive ways with
which one can cope with the hypothetical nothingness that
is existential anxiety.

3.1. Impact on Daily Functioning

Finally, victims of existential anxiety may be less likely to partake in religion, which is a potential source of comfort for individuals who find death anxiety to be important. Current research holds that religion, even in secular forms, reduces anxiety and provides a more optimistic worldview which can promote mental health and well-being. Overall, existential anxiety may be maladaptive and/or facilitate the development of other negative states which can contribute to mental health disorders or impact health in an adverse manner. In general, this level of worry. Individuals in a sample have reported moderate severity depression, anxiety symptoms, and suicidality in connection with existential anxiety.

One of the central themes of existential anxiety is the different ways it can impact an individual's day-to-day life. The impact is generally negative and maladaptive in nature. For anxious individuals, the thoughts and worries about existence and meaning can pervade one's thoughts, which detracts or consumes mental energy and leisure time that can be used for other forms of healthy meditation or relaxation. Existential anxiety has also been found to be tied to a crisis of meaning and loss of life purpose, which are important components of feelings of satisfaction, contentment, and overall well-being. For human beings, feelings of satisfaction as well as activities and beliefs that connect the individual to a sense of broader purpose are integral components of what make life enjoyable and worth living. Though it is agreed that the preservation of culture and system self is not the centre of life, it is quite clear and widely accepted that engagement and meaning in life is at least one motivational schema influencing many people and has been part of many different psychological traditions.

Even in less severe forms, the more pivotal the meaning system that is destroyed, the more chaotic emotional and cognitive experience is likely to be, and concomitant levels of panic and fear respondingly traumatic. This can lead to substances being used to mask emotional pain.

Research has also shown a strong relationship between anxiety, including existential anxiety, and excessive risk-taking, including an increasing vulnerability to substance abuse.

There is evidence of meaningful comorbidity between existential anxiety and anxiety disorders.

A relationship between existential anxiety and depression is well-documented, and a group of researchers have sought to highlight what they considered to be differences in the quality of these experiences.

If untreated, existential anxiety may intersect with other comorbid forms of psychological distress, aggravating their presentation and their course:

Unlike major depressive disorder and anxiety disorders, existential anxiety cannot be understood or easily distinguished in terms of biological or psychological etiologies. However, existential anxiety likely exacerbates these conditions, leading to treatment-challenging symptoms and/or presentations. For example, a person with pre-existing mental health difficulties may feel utterly demoralized (in an existential sense) as a result of a relationship breakdown and struggle to cling to a sense of life's ultimate worth or meaning. In these ways, preventing or addressing existential angst could be clinically important.

Before outlining our therapeutic approach, it is necessary to consider the role of existential anxiety within the broader mental health landscape, to differentiate it from other mental health conditions.

4. Therapeutic Approaches to Addressing Existential Anxiety

In conceptualizing the therapeutic approaches discussed, it has been considered that the most effective methods to address existential anxiety are those that seek to work with the individual in turn and enable them to increase their ability to cope. It has been noted that existential therapies can help with coping regarding the putative existence of a universal annihilation. Indeed, it is proposed that all forms of philosophically based therapies enable the individual to cope with the existence of their own potential oblivion. In essence, these therapeutic approaches assume that a form of psycho-education will assist the individual in understanding reality and dealing with the potential lack of an afterlife. These existential therapies, however, do not directly address the unique form of existential anxiety identified in this conceptualization.

There are several therapeutic approaches centered on addressing the experience of existential anxiety. The most notable of these approaches is existential therapy. In existential therapy, the aim is to explore and make sense of the client's experience. In addition to existential therapy-based approaches, several cognitive-behavioral therapy techniques have been adapted to address existential anxiety. Although these therapeutic approaches are not explicitly based upon terror management and do not explicitly measure death-awareness, it is possible that certain therapeutic techniques may lead to greater death-denial and higher DMT ratings. Regardless, based on previous findings, it is believed that these approaches may be insufficient, as it is important to create tailored interventions to reduce terror, which has implications for overall psychological well-being.

4. Therapeutic Approaches for Addressing Existential Anxiety

4.1. Existential Therapy

Practitioners of this tradition are less concerned with institutionalizing treatment and more interested in challenging the individual to embark on a philosophical examination of their own existence. By elucidating existential problems with the living of their life and guidance towards a more solid acceptance of their ultimate fates, existential psychotherapists hope to reveal the resilient existential problems within any specifically traumatic event. In this way, the existential therapist encourages patients to "suffer the anxiety of full human awareness, allowing the energy it releases to point the way to live more fully" in the light of one's personal fate. Some in this tradition have even compared existential therapy with an individual philosophical analysis of one's life such as that undertaken by Socrates. It provides a space where an individual's ultimate concerns can be clarified, and where the philosopher can begin at last to hone not just their philosophy but the life which it motivates.

Existential therapy, on the other hand, begins by asserting that the existential problems are particularly egregious aspects of human life. Its central concern lies in our awakening to the fact that our lives have no intrinsic meanings, and recognizing the resultant paralysis. Our intimate relationships, professional concerns, dreams, values, and ambitions – all turn out to be mere "habits of meaning" that we cultivate to comfort ourselves. We are fundamentally "thrown" into the world, without knowing why and without the possibility of recall, alone and free to invest our lives in any way we see fit. We are free to give meaning to our existence, but meaningfulness is not a feature of the world as such. As such, existential therapy is predominantly concerned with revealing the existential problems that traumatic events are nested within and counseling the individual towards a more total acceptance of the unique concerns of their existence.

4.2. Cognitive-Behavioral Therapy (CBT) Techniques

For some individuals, existential issues can also lead to increased feelings of distress. Research-supported treatments for anxiety, such as cognitive-behavioral methods, are amenable to addressing specific thought patterns and behaviors that contribute to existential anxiety. The use of such techniques can result in the empowerment and increased self-efficacy described above, while also alleviating the distress associated with existential emotions. Ellis (1962) and Beck (1976) proposed that it is not the directly relieving of an existential crisis that is most beneficial, but rather an adaptive restructuring of thought patterns and behaviors that would lead by inference to the dissolving of the crisis. CBT techniques are, in general, instrumental and practical. That is, the emphasis is not oriented toward finding and interpreting the ultimate causes and factors of a presenting problem and making a change over time based on insights gained in treatment. CBT typically addresses what an individual is doing now that might be contributing to their difficulties, and upon theory-driven strategies, toward overcoming those difficulties.

Cognitive-behavioral therapy (CBT) techniques: A number of recent works propose integrating existential philosophy with research-supported treatment modalities, such as cognitive-behavioral techniques, to help individuals with existential anxiety. Construct and Narrative Therapy is designed to help clients construct a more authentic story to inform their conceptions of the world and of their place within it. The primary aim of the following works is to address the maladaptive thought patterns that may be associated with existential issues, while also empowering individuals to adopt existentialist themes in a way that is life-enhancing.

5. Utilizing Existential Anxiety for Personal Growth

Existential dilemmas, however, also contain a meaningful dimension and may therefore also contain a positive aspect, which is to enhance the otherwise implicit personal engagement with life. The encounter with incompatibilities gives rise to a cure called "existential anxiety": it is self-organizing frustration and can be filled by the person if a behavioral and meaningful accommodation becomes more difficult. The individual may be able to have a better overall understanding and possibly increase consciousness by mastering the existential anxiety. An encounter with the incompatibility through existential anxiety may have the potential to cure. If the individual succeeds in mastering his anxiety, he may have a greater understanding of his situation and a foundation of personal growth. In particular, Storr stressed that creative endurance through existential anxiety is of immense importance since anxiety is a prominent feature of artists throughout history. Implication has often advised giving people more freedom to linger with their anxiety and have a responsibility for leading to new stability.

The human existence essentially involves issues that cannot be answered conclusively: we refer to common life experience as "existential dilemmas." Having no satisfying solution increases psychic tension and is often accompanied by deep discomfort. How do people learn to live with this pain? Humans can communicate their experiences and fears to other individuals, while animals can attempt to flee or rescue themselves, relax, be comfortable, have a good meal, or control something. As Freud has emphasized, human life as a whole is not a comfortable arrangement that can always be changed when we have learned to be happy. Any human being must face at least 3 deadly states: life can end, diseases and aging, and other termination agents can be encountered. Humanity must learn to live with effort, pain, or existential uncertainty.

5.1. Finding Meaning and Purpose

The content of introspective philosophy and psychology is
as boundless and varied as human experience. Accordingly,
the following is not a survey of every such insight gleamed,
but is instead intended to provide, at several points in this
book, a taste of the ideas and the depths of introspective
inquiry. In what follows, note that I am not espousing a
particular philosophical or psychological point of view,
whether implicitly or explicitly. The trials and sufferings of
life are innumerable, and what makes one person thrive
can make another's spirit wilt. And yet there is complexity
and depth. There is an opportunity to make friends with
the fleeting nature of existence, to press its difficulties and
pain into the service of creativity, compassion, and
wisdom.

Existential anxiety presents the opportunity to explore and
find meaning, purpose, and sometimes even spiritual truth.
If we can embrace the subjective, emotional, personal
dimension of our seconds, minutes, and hours on a level
deeper than any of our technologies yet reach, we can learn
profound things about ourselves and our relationships to
others and the world. Such a process—an exploration at
greater depth, appreciating many different ways meaning
gets living out of bed—is at the heart of existential
philosophy and counseling. As we will explore next,
existential anxiety can be a difficult, sometimes impossible
block to feeling grounded enough to embark on such
efforts. However, as will also see, existential struggle can

yield profound existential growth if we know how to leverage it wisely.

5.2. Cultivating Resilience

It is very difficult to know ourselves with certainty, to remain present in the moment even when the next moment might bring terrible news. It is critical evidence of the human spirit that so many people do. This section will discuss work in progress on the training of therapists and other healthcare professionals to support people in their existential journey. Master classes have been run in person and webinar format to support therapists in the critical work of facing our own existential fears and capacities. Although it is a cliché to use the term "inner resources" in this context, many people are remarkably resilient, experiencing growth in personal development and relationships, given the necessary support. An implicit false message in society is to treat grief as a mental health issue, a message that inevitably becomes damaging to grief. Grief is painful. Grief is universal.

In addition to the adaptive responses, inner strengths, and values that can emerge when confronting the existential challenges in this therapeutic approach, another critical plenary theme was the implications for building resilience from an MLE perspective. By reflecting on how existential attitudes and self-regulation techniques can help to manage and mitigate existential anxiety, it is not intended to "medicalize" or minimize the challenges presented by the "accumulation of untenable grief". The aim is neither to propose a magic bullet that helps patients "recover", nor to ignore, deny, or bypass the existential sources of distress and anxiety. Rather, the focus is on how people can develop existential resilience in the face of these challenges, as they do not know the outcome.

6. Case Studies and Practical Applications

For the near future research, it would be of great interest to perform a focus group analysis where participants of the proposed SAEP program could be given the freedom to discuss their insights and thoughts. This would doubtlessly require a follow-up program to ensure the group has maintained the perspectives and insights. The relation between the case study contents and underlying axioms remains unexamined and will need to be investigated in future research.

This paper has attempted to depict a philosophical exploration and therapeutic approach to existential anxiety. What began as a conceptual investigation into our ability to deal with alarm, distress, and anguish culminated in the theoretical exploration of an adequate framework and effective interventions to address such distress. Using a case-study methodology, it was shown how the proposed therapeutic approach allowed the participants to reinterpret the alarm-inducing existential event in a constitutive way. The participants no longer viewed their distressing event as a traumatic or pathological occurrence but as part of their unfolding meaning. From the results, it can furthermore be hypothesized that the participants now understand and can read the trigger that initially caused their distress. This has installed them with constitutionally endowed tools to better appreciate, understand, and cultivate their embedded worlds.

Introduction

6.1. Real-life Examples of Existential Anxiety

The mental and physical suffering outlined in these quotes, each in response to the question of how do you experience existential doubts or anxiety?, illustrates frustrations and fears which occur on multiple levels: the fear of losing oneself, fears about what we have become, repulsion about the fact that we are so easily reassimilated into nature, because an uncertainty about the actual state of things, also unknown what this might lead to, and finally a loneliness, because such deep metaphysical questions are less often shared in the public sphere. The narratives in this section each show us how people grapple with existential doubts – it is an attempt to put people's psychic suffering into a broader narrative, an attempt to, as Bollnow writes, "bridge the gap between formalistic metaphysical problems and the concreteness of experience". This, indeed, directly allows the therapist (the recipient of these narratives) to interact at a level that closer to the other and offers a window to develop analytic insights. If, as Yalom claims, "Many patients cannot learn to search for meaning until psychotherapy offers them the chance to experience their therapist as a meaningful person", real-life examples of existential anxieties must also offer an enhanced reflective space in terms of the therapeutical approach.

Example 4: "Existence to me screamed: I am more than this. We are all more than this. We need to somehow weave ourselves into our very existence, no matter the actual cost. We are somehow more than what we have, but at the same time others are unnerved at the thought of us having nothing."

Before we progress, however, it might be insightful to follow three examples of existential struggles informed from real therapy sessions, as observed in our clinical practice. In these examples, three unique life narratives – a feeling of always sticking out, a sudden out-of-body experience, and a fear of dying and becoming reassimilated by nature – are given in response to the question of how do you experience existential doubts or anxiety? The narratives, though unique, all provide a sense of the multifaceted ways in which the idea of existence causes despair.

6.2. Therapeutic Interventions and Outcomes

All seeded interventions were effective in some way for the general population within particular sectors as well in ameliorating the interpersonal, workplace, education, and clinical issues highlighted in the stress models as describing our existential destruction. Indeed, beyond interpersonal and clinical stress as outcomes, for the healthy population, all treatments were effective in improving the mental as well as well-being symptoms linked with the psycho-complex adaptation systems controlled by our HPA anxiety systems, such as improvements in mood, wellbeing, dread/despair, and physical symptoms. In addition, the chronological and longitudinal research studies demonstrate the heightened effectiveness of decreasing anxiety and increasing quality of life.

The last four sections of the tables give us some evidence for the effectiveness of some of these general as well as topic-specific interventions in the general population. Rathnow et al. (2012) proved that the effectiveness of general CBT and mindfulness-based treatment is particularly effective in treating distress, but also the specific treatment of the trauma that activated the anxiety is ameliorating the sleep-related (i.e., non-existential) PTSD symptoms (such as fear of trauma-specific related stimuli and activities) in (women) inmates.

To date, there are relatively few therapeutic interventions for existential anxiety, and outcomes are generally short term because of the endpoints of many psychological and psychiatric counseling services. Nevertheless, there are some approaches that may have practical implications and that may also allow some generalization of changing attitudes in increasing despair, loneliness, or meaninglessness found in many countries as pointed out by Wood et al. (2010) (also Pillai and Howell, 2016).

7. Conclusion and Future Directions

Research into the nature of existential concerns is still in its infancy. While we have laid some preliminary groundwork in connection to how it may be possible to alleviate the suffering caused by our existential malaise, much more empirical work needs to be conducted before we are able to propose a comprehensive theory of how we might be able to alleviate this type of distress. For instance, although we have proposed that CBT and meaning-centered therapies might be able to help assuage some components of existential distress by directly challenging or helping to replace some of the negative, fearful thoughts that this can lead to, it remains to be studied systematically what causes and maintains these distressing cognitions. In addition, empirical work has still to be conducted to examine the validity of our division of existential distress into different categories, and into how these groups of concerns interrelate. Only when we examine some of these crucial questions will we be properly positioned to lay the foundations for a comprehensive approach to addressing the multitudinous aspects of existential suffering.

Fears of death and the suffering that follows are a natural part of life. However, these fears can become a source of anxiety that can render life unbearable. In this paper, we have drawn from both psychological and philosophical literature to develop a new typology of existential anxiety. We have shown that existential anxiety can cover a range of experiences and can result from various thoughts and beliefs about death. And we have sought out how these different aspects of existential anxiety can be integrated to present a comprehensive way of understanding the various ways in which people respond to the idea of their own mortality. While this overview presents a novel way at unpacking issues of existential concern, a lot of work in this area remains to be done. We hope our representations of different aspects of existential anxiety can be of use in furthering our understanding of these concerns, and in developing new approaches to alleviating existential despair.